Caregiving

Church and Family Together

OLDER ADULT ISSUES SERIES

The Office of Older Adult Ministry of the Presbyterian
Church (U.S.A.) and Geneva Press are grateful for the
generous gifts of many individuals, congregations, and
organizations that helped make possible the publication
of this series.

Caregiving
Church and Family Together

Marty Richards

Published for the Office of Older Adult Ministry,
A Ministry of the General Assembly Council,
Presbyterian Church (U.S.A.)

Geneva Press
Louisville, Kentucky

Contents

Preface

Mary Smith, sixty, is a member of First Presbyterian Church. She cares for her husband John, sixty-five, who has been struggling with Alzheimer's disease for five years. Three years ago Mary quit her job as a nurse at the local hospital to become John's full-time caregiver. Formerly very active in her congregation, Mary now only attends Sunday services on rare occasions. She is thankful that the church's parish nurse has been faithfully supportive to her and her husband. John's care needs are increasing, and Mary is struggling with planning for his future care.

John Andrews is ninety-two. Three years ago, his wife of sixty years, Anna, eighty-nine, suffered a stroke. He has been her full-time caregiver since then. He had never cooked before her stroke, but is now proud of the cooking skills he has learned. John has Parkinson's disease and his illness is making it more and more difficult to care for his wife. Despite the fact that he and his wife have been life-long members of John Knox Presbyterian Church, he has refused offers from the Volunteer Respite Ministry of his church to come for a few hours each week and provide relief for him.

Susan Jones is fifty-three. She lives in Seattle. Her mom, who is eighty-three, lives in Chicago and has been an active member of Bethany Presbyterian Church.

Susan's mother is becoming very frail as a result of heart problems and chronic pain associated with compression fractures. She also struggles with poor vision related to glaucoma. Although her sister Karen, fifty-five, cares daily for her mom, Susan is very concerned about the quality of Karen's care for her mother. She often feels out of the loop and wishes that the church would do more to support her sister and her mom.

Jim Adams is forty. He and his wife Carol, active members of Westminster Presbyterian Church, have moved his mom, who is seventy-five, into their home because she is dying of brain cancer. Because he works each day, his wife has taken over the full-time caregiving. The stresses of his mom's illness are affecting his marital relationship, and at times he has found himself yelling at his mom when her behavior seems bizarre. When people at church on Sunday morning ask how he is doing he replies, "I am fine, just fine."

All of these people are members of our churches. Each finds him- or herself in a caregiving relationship. All struggle with difficult caregiving issues. Each is dealing with the situation in his or her own unique way. Each might benefit from assistance from the congregation along the caregiving journey. Are Mary, John, Susan, and Jim members of your congregation? How can you reach out to them? This book addresses caregiving and the church's response to caregivers' needs.

Introduction

We are caregivers at different times throughout our lives. Caring for children when they are babies and as they grow is expected. For the most part, people look forward to the challenges of that process. They may plan ahead and encourage extended family members to walk that path with them in the exciting time of watching a child grow.

Many of us will face caregiving in the middle and later years of our lives as well. But this time it is different. Most of us don't really think that we will be caring for our partners, parents, grandparents, or other aged relatives as they struggle with disabling conditions. And what a big surprise it is to face issues in caring for a spouse struggling with ill health. So, even though in our minds we might have thought, "It could happen to me," most of us are overwhelmed when we find ourselves in the caring role.

This book is about caregiving to those with disabilities in the middle and later years. Some issues faced by most caregivers and care receivers are universal; some are unique. There are overwhelming challenges with which to cope, but there are also compensations. There is no cookbook for handling every concern, but some suggestions will be offered that you can adapt to your own situation.

In over thirty years of social work practice, and in my personal life, I have met caregivers who have shared with me the experience of being involved in the day-to-day process of assisting someone: the joys and the struggles— the grief and the hope. They have taught me about love, forgiveness, and patience. Adaptation, creativity, and coping have been their themes. They are like the people I introduced in the preface.

On the other hand, caregivers have helped me understand what comes into play when the caring gets to be too much. They have taught me important truths about what happens when, for the sake of care receiver and caregiver, the daily care must be assumed by another person, agency, or institution. And these committed people have opened my eyes to the problems that arise from macrosystem issues such as demographic factors, federal and state policies, or regulations that work against aging families. The caregivers and care receivers that I have known are special people of commitment and courage, and I owe them thanks for being my mentors. It is my hope that some of what they have taught me, information that I will share through this book, can assist you in your own caregiving, or help you to stand shoulder to shoulder with those who find themselves in that role. Neighbors and members of your congregation need help in caregiving. You yourself may be struggling with such concerns.

Caregiving can be both an opportunity and a burden, often a long journey with no end in sight. Serious illness changes how family life evolves. For example, the former breadwinner may become a very dependent person. The housewife may have to take on financial accounts that had previously been managed by her husband. Intimate care tasks may change the rules of how to act in the family. While giving gentle care, there may be a chance to exchange feelings of love, warmth, and support. For example, giving back to a parent who has nurtured you as a child can be very rewarding. Estranged siblings may learn new ways to relate and may pull together to assure the provision of good quality of life for a parent.

At the same time, these same tasks can cause extreme burdens. This is especially true when the care receiver has a dementia or other problem that causes them to forget their caregiver. A previously independent care receiver may express anger toward a caregiver while basic hygiene needs are being met. Frustration in this experience revolves around a feeling of indignity, and is sometimes played out in hurtful ways toward the caregiver. Sibling concerns left on the back burner for years may bubble up again during long-term caregiving and create difficulties for everyone.

Caregiving gives opportunities for reciprocity between generations. Such give-and-take is important for the integrity of all in caregiving roles. As one generation has cared for another in the past, there is the chance for giving back, concretely and emotionally. There is much that can be shared between those giving care and those receiving care: love, concern, humor, and survival skills. This is consistent with the Christian tradition of interdependency, of giving and receiving care, and of loving one another even as Christ loved.

The church can support persons struggling with such issues. In communities of faith, clergy and laypersons alike can walk alongside those on the difficult road of caring. For helpers to really help, they must also be open to the gift of learning from caregivers *and* care receivers. And they must be willing to listen to stories of emotional pain and sadness, and not make pronouncements based on some formula for what "ought to be." What *is* for a particular family needs to be heard. Each caregiving situation is unique; each family constellation makes decisions based on what is best for them. There is no one-size-fits-all formula or solution. The ideas here are shared in the hope that they can facilitate the church's response to assisting those who are caregivers. Aiding caregivers means carrying out the church's mandate to heal, reconcile, and bind up wounds, and to minister to the needs of the sick. Ministry is *with* elders and their families not *to* them.

1 Some Basic Foundations

Older members of families have gifts and face challenges. Understanding this can go a long way in uplifting family members in their roles. Several basic premises about family caregiving can set the stage for how support might be given most effectively. The community of faith needs to understand these foundations if ministry to caregivers is to be truly effective.

The Family Is a System

The family is a system, and it is important to older adults. Even those who are estranged from family, or who have outlived other family members, will recount family stories and will express loss of connection. Family is the place where people learn to trust or not trust others, and to understand how to live in relationship. Families can serve as lifelines to their members. While these ideas may seem self-evident, some programs to help older adults operate as if elders and disabled adults live in a vacuum.

People may define "family" in a variety of ways. Different ethnic and cultural groups may be more or less inclusive of who belongs in the family circle, who bears responsibility for caring for disabled members, who should make decisions, and who should be caregivers. Obviously some very clear legal definitions about what constitutes family exist. For purposes of this book, families are those who provide nurture and support (emotional, material, spiritual) over time. Such persons may or may not be related by blood or marriage. The family includes those persons one can count on when there is a need for very practical assistance or a listening ear. Or, in the words of a one-hundred-year-old friend, it encompasses "those who love us with our warts." Within such a definition, persons from the faith community are family. Caregivers *are* important for those who need help. As each definition of family is unique, so too is the family's view of caregiving. Both those giving care and those receiving care are members of congregations. There is a need to keep in touch with both, affirming the special situation in which they find themselves.

Caregiving across the Generations
Caregiving affects many generations, young and old. There is a need to balance the needs of all within the aging family, as challenges abound. Because the number of those sixty-five and older is growing so rapidly, and because that group tends to have many chronic care conditions that limit their lives, family members will be providing more care. While there are more people growing to advanced old age, there are not as many in the adult children age category to be carers. There will be fewer people available to be caregivers as women, traditional caregivers, have entered the workplace. Families of four and five generations facing caregiving dilemmas will be more

common due to increased longevity of the oldest old (*Profile of Older Americans*, 1997).

Questions of quality of life will be raised, and there is no right or wrong answer. But keeping the balance for all generations in caregiving is important. Many ethical questions need to be raised and explored. Pastoral counselors, parish nurses, Stephen ministers, and others can listen to such questions. Adult education classes can provide the springboard for discussions. To empower caregivers to be supportive to those they care about, all generations in the aging family benefit from nurture from the church. Even the youngest persons in a family may provide companionship and loving support to a disabled person. The child needs an explanation of illness in ways that are understandable in order to decrease fears and increase interaction. Often there is a special bond between elder and child, and support can be offered without strings attached.

Supporting Caregivers
Persons in the caregiving role do better when they perceive that they are not alone; that others understand their problems. Isolation can be a concern, and as the person they care for becomes more frail, it may seem that many, even long-term friends, pull away. Caregivers may have the sense that they are not cared about. Those from the church may not be comfortable with an ill person. There are several reasons for this. A most basic reason is that a person confronts his or her own mortality, and realizes that he or she could be mentally or physically challenged one

day, every time he or she encounters someone who is ill. This can be scary, and people can be troubled by such thoughts, which can then become impediments to being comfortable when visiting the ill. Also, visitors may not be able to cope with the fact that someone they have known as vital and healthy, a deacon or Sunday school teacher, for example, is now a frail elder. People need to be approached as they are at that moment. For the church to be supportive, members need to examine their personal issues about disability. Being available to the sick and to those who care about them means confronting one's own mortality.

Being able to honestly share concerns with a good listener can be a gift to a caregiver's sanity, and can also prevent potential situations of caregiver burnout. Clergy and laypersons will not have all the answers, but they do need to be able to do some difficult listening. Church members can be part of a network of help for caregivers. Practical ways to decrease feelings of isolation might include respite care and regular check-in calls for the caregiver and care receiver.

Kinds of Care
Caregiving takes many forms, but is most often thought of as those who provide hands-on care. Some family members may be caregivers in other ways, offering trips to the doctor, shopping, phone calls, and other services. Some may be long-distance caregivers. All in the family system could benefit from faith-community help. Examples of

such assistance might include adult education classes where caregiving information is shared, and words from the pulpit about what it means to give and receive care or how it feels to be independent or dependent. All in the family struggling with the dependencies of a disabled person may need spiritual, hands-on, and emotional care.

A Changing Demographic

While each family system is unique, it is affected by the demographics and policies of the larger society. Future projections predict that the number of elders will increase as baby boomers advance to retirement age. The decreasing birth and mortality rates will mean that there will be more elders cared for by fewer persons in the adult children ages. This will influence the aid that families will be able to offer. What is known about caregiving today and what will be true in the future may be different. New paradigms for caregiving may need to be developed. Congregations have a responsibility to confront all ages with the realization that they are aging. Concerns for justice between generations should also be discussed within the context of the congregational community.

Economic and Political Policies

Economic and political policies influence families' abilities to provide eldercare. Two general policies that affect families include family leave and Medicare. They influence where persons should be cared for, who will be doing the caring, and how that caring will be reimbursed. A reality is that a person may have to work full time for financial survival, which leaves precious little time to spend with a loved one. Even if that person chooses to leave a paying job to care for a disabled family member, in this country (unlike many others) they will usually not be compensated. And there may not be any assurance that the job will be there when they want to return to employment. This may be true even after years of service. The federal Family Leave Act has alleviated some concerns related to this, but not all. Because of these factors, a logical family carer may not be able to do hands-on caring. At times, caregivers are blamed for not caring, when in reality they are caught between such rocks and hard places. To assist caregivers, churches need to be aware of how policy issues affect families. Issues of justice and fairness can be considered. Understanding these macrosystem concerns is crucial to appreciating all that caregiving families face.

Family Life Cycles
Families have their own life cycles. Historical events of family life do affect what happens in caregiving. What is happening in society at large also has an effect. Intergenerational relationships influence all family members throughout life. There is a circular correlation between relationships over time and how eldercare is provided. If there have been estrangements or unresolved conflicts, there may be difficulties in caregiving. Without interventions, there are situations where generations who have been abused as young persons abuse a frail elder. The

community of faith can perform an important safety valve function, and pastoral care with caregivers may include the need for working on issues of forgiveness. Support offered to carers might help prevent another generation of family dysfunction.

2   Family Dynamics

The way a family gives care is influenced by the family dynamics that have been in place prior to persons becoming caregivers and care receivers. These processes remain at work when a family faces caring for someone with physical problems or dementia.

Family Roles

Family roles are a big part of family dynamics. Roles evolve over time and are selected or thrust on people early in the family's development, then remain over a family life span. The reasons why roles were assigned may be forgotten, but families note, "It's the way it's always been." Sometimes roles developed over time as persons dealt with functional changes. Roles can be reexamined and renegotiated in the later years as families face challenges.

Many roles are biological. For example, one is a mother, daughter, father, son, or grandmother by virtue of birth. Such biological roles also have psychological and psychosocial implications. A grandmother is "supposed to" do certain things, act in a special way, or experience particular feelings. And these biological roles may influence who should be a caregiver.

Historical roles are played over time. Acting as the

matriarch or patriarch of the family are examples of such roles. These roles require respect from younger family members. Matriarchs and patriarchs are often repositories of family stories, and they dictate the way that families do things. Historical roles can also have negative connotations. The black sheep or estranged child are roles that some have played over a lifetime. When an elder needs care, these roles can be raised again and create pain for the family unit.

Functional roles are important, and assist persons in tangible ways. These family roles that help elders include "Mr./Ms. Fixit" (doing basic household projects), the "switchboard operator" (getting people mobilized), and caregiver. The "pot stirrer," on the other hand, is the member who operates in a way that runs counter to other family members and can create difficulties as plans are made. These concrete functional roles can mean the difference between someone staying at home or needing outside help in the home or in an institution.

Relational roles are also crucial in keeping a family together. The person who is the legacy giver or legacy keeper keeps the family history of facts, emotions, strains, and successes and passes them from generation to generation. A social organizer plans special events for holidays, birthdays, and reunions. Their challenge is to keep an elder an integral part of the family unit; a large concern when an elder struggles with frailty or dementia.

Examining roles and the tasks related to them can help caregivers. People may take on new roles. An adult daughter may bathe her elderly mom. Sometimes a caregiver has taken on too much and becomes a martyr. Families may need some third-party help (counselor or minister for example) to explore family roles. Lustbader and Hooyman in *Taking Care of Aging Family Members* (1994, p. 77) offer ideas for looking at these roles and tasks, and give practical steps for renegotiating them.

Family Rules

Family rules are another part of family dynamics. They govern the way that families share information and caring. Whether unspoken or clearly articulated, they are powerful predictors of why families do things in certain ways. Rules may evolve from religious or philosophical beliefs; they may be part of a cultural imperative, or they may simply be derived from an individual family's perspective based in family history. Some may immobilize a family even when they are not articulated. Those families who have struggled with addictions over time may have developed a rule about not accurately perceiving a situation. Such a rule is counterproductive in trying to care for a person who is struggling with memory losses. Rules that affect families include: "This family cares for its own," "We save for a rainy day," "This family fights with each other, but don't try to help us, or we'll turn on you," and "Don't air dirty linen in public." Caregivers may delay asking for assistance because it is not compatible with the rule of "caring for one's own."

Since many rules about caring in the family are based on

theological perspectives, adult education classes, and especially Bible studies, might be developed to assist all in examining these concerns. In pastoral care situations, exploring such rules may help families understand what is motivating their behaviors.

Family Secrets
Family secrets also play a role in family dynamics. These are the events or people known to some while withheld from others. Secrets include such things as abuse, incest, alcoholism, mental illness, infidelity, suicide, and adoption. These long-term issues may affect the quality of the caregiving provided and at times even who the caregiver might be. The abuse of a young daughter by her drunken father may make it very difficult for that adult child to care for him after a stroke. The church needs to be aware that these secrets exist at some level for most families. While not always spoken out loud, they may create difficulties in the caregiving situation. It is important to remember that concerns that are now openly discussed, such as mental illness and alcoholism, were taboo in the early lives of elders, and there may be great feelings of shame if they are revealed. There may be secrets in families where the process of forgiveness is needed.

These parts of family dynamics, roles, rules, and secrets are powerful factors in caregiving. They cannot be ignored by caregivers or the community of faith. In a general way they might be explored in adult education settings. Personal concerns may require pastoral counseling or support from the parish nurse.

3   Practical Concerns

Most caregiving in this country is done in a family context with variation in how this is provided. Society has been slow to affirm the unsung heroes who day in and day out give hours of care. Because of the lack of acknowledgment, a sense of isolation increases for many caregivers.

Women are the primary caregivers at all stages of family life. Traditionally women have been socialized to be nurturers, and this has been reinforced by the church. By default, rules and expectations define caregiving for elders and the disabled as a woman's role. Women live longer than men. And many women in the current cohort of older adults marry men who are the same age or older. These demographic trends help explain why so many women care for disabled spouses and aging parents. Although caregiving is primarily a women's issue, this is not to discount the work that men do as caregivers. However, women are expected to do it, while men are affirmed for the special contributions they make when they are in the caregiving role. A question that could be asked by a congregation is, "How do we affirm our caregivers, especially the women, in our church?"

What is it like to be a caregiver? While it varies, communities of faith can become aware of caregiving's practical aspects. An understanding of some basic issues can go a long way in equipping the church to be truly compassionate toward both caregiver and care receiver. If a congregation desires to know what is needed by their own caregivers, they should ask them, listen to their concerns, and then put any suggestions into practice.

Relationships are altered in the caregiving and care receiving experience. Physical losses and changes are many. The onset of an illness such as a stroke has obvious devastating features. There are more basic physical changes that can also be difficult: changes in hearing, vision, taste, and mobility. All can decrease a person's ability to take care of him or herself.

For care receivers, social changes may include loss of a long-term partner and intimacy as they have known it, loss of close friends, loss of a pet, loss of ability, loss of income, and loss of identity in society. Ultimately the loss of one's own life looms as a major concern. Care receivers often report feeling alone and trapped in their situation. These changes affect how a person perceives receiving care as well.

There are also losses and changes for caregivers. It is difficult for the spouse of forty, fifty, or sixty years to watch a loved one deteriorate. For long-term partners loss of intimacy can be devastating. Another very difficult loss occurs when a parent can't be the parent to an adult child. This creates major changes in the relationship and children grieve.

Physical care is an overwhelming part of providing aid to a disabled person. Lifting, bathing, feeding, and toileting are some of the tasks that a person may carry out in providing for a person with limitations. These jobs, added to general household tasks, are physically exhausting and emotionally draining. At times, family caregivers could benefit from receiving help to carry out such tasks. Some steadfastly feel that they must do all the work themselves to fulfill the requirements of loving their care receiver. Adding to this stress, there are some care receivers who complain that their carer does not do a task correctly. Not getting affirmation from a care receiver can be very demoralizing. The church can "reframe" with caregivers about how they perceive their responsibilities. It is a sign of strength to seek help, but many have been taught over the years that it indicates weakness. Congregations can remind caregivers they are not weak when they request assistance. One stressed caregiver learned these lessons the hard way after suffering a stroke. He shared this bit of wisdom at a workshop: "Even Superman is Clark Kent most of the time!" This is a useful message for all caregivers.

Both caregivers and care receivers struggle with dependency. Many have prided themselves on being fiercely independent throughout life. The thought of informing others about the difficulties they face is distasteful. Dependency on another for basic care needs can feel demeaning to a care receiver. It is emotionally painful for a care receiver to know that he or she cannot, or has only limited ways, to give back to the caregiver. An analogy might be apt here. Many grew up in a time when a friend brought over a casserole as a sign of love and concern when there was sickness or bereavement. One would never think of returning that dish without making cookies or putting something else in the bowl to say thanks. It was the expected hospitable behavior. So think about how someone would feel if they only received casseroles every day without being able to reciprocate in some way. They would experience a loss of self-esteem. People receiving care may feel this decreasing self-esteem when they can't give back in any way. And this can be true even when the caregivers are kind and compassionate. Creating ways for care receivers to give back is important. It may be as simple as having them tell their story of survival.

Some receiving care get angry about it. That anger is often expressed toward the person who delivers care, the very person to whom they are closest emotionally. Such lashing out may take on a very personal flavor and is devastating to a person trying to do their best. Caregivers may need to reframe anger. Usually it is not really directed at a caregiver, but at the situation in which a person finds him- or herself. Those receiving care become angry at caregivers precisely because they are family. Obviously there can be a great deal of variation in family experience. To be supportive, the church needs to grasp this reality. Wendy Lustbader's wonderful book, *Counting on Kindness: The Dilemmas of Dependency* (1994), explores this topic in some depth, and should be required reading for all in the religious community who would minister to caregivers and care receivers.

Caregivers may feel trapped by their loved one's need for care. Those assisting persons with Alzheimer's disease tell tales related to a lack of privacy, even to the point of being followed into the bathroom! Or they may be awakened several times at night to help a person who is scared or who may need to use the bathroom. Overwhelming exhaustion and fatigue set in. Some have talked about "the thirty-six-hour day" (Mace and Rabins, 1991). In these situations respite care can be a lifesaver. Giving the caregiver time away from twenty-four-hour-a-day responsibility pays dividends for mental health and for maintaining relationships. The church could provide volunteers to be with someone a few hours per week, giving caregivers a breather. Caregivers may also need a listening ear from a pastoral counselor, Stephen minister, or parish nurse so that they could honestly express frustrations without being judged.

Besides hands-on responsibilities, caregivers may worry about finances. Family income can be a concern if a caregiver leaves a job to provide fulltime care. Medical costs are high, and not all needs are covered by Medicare or private insurance. The caregiver may also feel hurt if it appears that there will be no money left to receive as a legacy, or even enough to pay for their very basic survival. Churches can have resource material available about financial services. Being able to make appropriate referrals to agencies can be crucial in ministry with caregivers. Tuning in to these concerns can help both church staff and lay visitors to be sensitive to those who struggle with financial concerns.

4   Feelings Families Face

In addition to the practical things with which they struggle, families may also have intense emotions when dealing
with issues related to a loved one's disability and resultant
caregiving requirements. Naming and talking about these
feelings goes a long way in enabling persons to continue
on the caregiving journey. It can be very therapeutic to
give voice to one's emotions. Otherwise they may inter-
nalize and fester. Just knowing that others face similar
concerns can be beneficial.

Caregivers and care receivers alike may have *fears*.
Some are stated out loud; many remain in their hearts
and minds. But spoken or not, both caregivers and carereceivers operate on them and make decisions based on
such fears. Fears can be related to what will happen to a
loved one if the caregiver is unable to provide enough care
or, ultimately, unable to continue providing care at all.
With so much negative press about long-term care facili-
ties and home care providers, caregivers may be fright-
ened. Underlying other fears may be the issue of whether
there will be enough money. For blood relatives of persons
with debilitating diseases (especially dementia), there can
be the question, "Could I be like this myself one day?"
Fears can immobilize caregivers, but being able to verbalize

the fears may help a person cope, even when it is not possible to solve all problems.

Other feelings revolve around *anger*, and there are many reasons for this. Anger is a normal feeling. Some caregivers feel that it is wrong to have such feelings and stuff the anger inside themselves. This is not healthy and can lead to depression. They need someone to listen to them as they talk it out; either one-on-one or in a support group. There can be anger at the debilitating illness for taking its toll, at having to be on duty all the time, at others in the family network who are not sharing the emotional or physical burden, or at watching financial resources ebb away. There also can be anger at the loss of plans and dreams such as unfulfilled hopes for retirement. One care receiver and his wife bought a camper before his retirement with plans to travel the country and enjoy their freedom. Before leaving his position, he suffered a stroke. Until it was sold a year later, the camper was parked in the driveway, a constant reminder of what might have been, and the couple had much understandable anger about that.

This kind of scenario is not uncommon. The change in lifestyle is very difficult even for the most devoted caregivers. Anger is normal, but those who do the caring need to express it in ways that are not harmful to the care receiver or to themselves. Taking a walk or talking to a friend who is a sounding board are examples of constructive ways to deal with anger. Persons from the faith community can provide the safety valves for anger's expression.

Listening to these issues without advice or judgment is crucial. Even examining what anger is from a Christian context can be helpful, as most have been taught to "stuff it."

Caregivers also almost universally feel *guilt* caused by current issues in the relationship or by past concerns. Guilt can be felt as a result of "sins of omission" and "sins of commission." Things that have been done, harsh words said, or times when one was less than charitable or lost their temper can create guilt. Even the need for respite, for time away, can cause a caregiver guilt. And there can be regret for things that were not done, such as the lost times to say "I love you," and the estranged relationships that were not healed. A loved one may have suffered a stroke, for example, making it impossible to work things out with him or her. It is important for guilt to be put into reasonable limits, so it does not immobilize the caregiver. Guilt rarely goes away completely, so it is not helpful to say to a caregiver, "You don't need to feel guilty about that." Caregivers do need to be reminded that they are doing the best that they can do. And there may be pastoral care opportunities for working through forgiveness issues with caregivers.

Sadness and *grief* underlie many caregiver feelings. For example, adult children may grieve the loss of the parent as they knew him or her before a stroke. A spouse may grieve the loss of intimacy and companionship when a partner struggles with Alzheimer's disease. Caregivers may grieve the loss of the way of life they have known, and may feel very sad over the loss of a planned future. Anticipatory grief can also be an especially difficult concern as one deals with the things that he or she knows are coming, such as selling a house to conserve expenses or amputating a limb due to circulatory problems.

The uncertainty of situations can also arouse feelings of sadness or grief. A person might be caring for a loved one in cancer's final stages. The dying person may be slowly but surely leaving this world but still be physically present. Grief can be overwhelming and needs to be identified and shared. Tears can be a healthy release, and sometimes just being with someone as they cry can be balm. Those who minister from the faith community can encourage caregiver tears to flow for healing. The church with its teachings about life and death is in a unique position to comfort those coping with sadness and grief. Ministry provides words and actions of love and concern.

Helplessness and *hopelessness* can overwhelm and are experienced as a feeling that nothing can change to improve a situation. The situation can be perceived as being too much, and that can be debilitating, and reflect the end of hope. *Loss of control* and *powerlessness* are related issues. For some there is a helpless feeling in the loss of all personal identity except as caregiver. Being able to take one step at a time is a crucial skill for ameliorating these feelings. When a person sees success in small events like a care receiver being able to wash his own face, it can yield big benefits emotionally. The church can be a connector, helping persons to connect with advocacy groups such as the Alzheimer's Association or support groups. Being involved with such groups can be empowering and can decrease the perceptions of helplessness and hopelessness experienced by caregivers.

Probably the most difficult emotions to deal with are those related to *ambivalence*. Love for the care receiver and dislike for the illness coexist in an internal psychological tug of war. An example that illustrates this frustration is the question of whether to continue to care for someone alone or to seek additional assistance. People can go back and forth in the assessment of their loved one's condition. There are issues of smothering versus necessary protection. Often a caregiver does not accurately perceive a loved one's condition and lives in denial because it is too painful to realize the loved one's limits. Ambivalence exists around how independent a person can be, when a person has a right to fail, and when the person needs to be closely monitored for safety.

Embarrassment can be experienced by caregivers coping with the unpredictable or socially unacceptable behaviors associated with some illnesses. Care receivers can be embarrassed. A person who has had a stroke might be uncomfortable about paralysis or drooling. Caregivers embarrassed by a person's losses might try to cover for this by not going to church or other social gatherings with their loved one, or by discouraging friends and those from the faith community from visiting. These actions can lead to increased isolation for the person with the illness and for the caregiver. While affirming the dignity of persons affected, illnesses need to be let out of the box so that others can respond appropriately and learn how to be more comfortable in the face of strange behaviors, especially when they happen at congregational events.

Despite all of these difficult feelings there also can be *laughter*, *love*, and *joy*. Families find strength in these feelings. Telling stories is a part of sharing these emotions. The care receiver, even a person with dementia, may be able to tell things that they remember from other parts of their lives. Someone needs to be available to witness their story. Humor can be a gift to sanity for caregivers and care receivers alike. Spiritual sharing is also important. Sometimes it is the simple act of singing a familiar hymn or praying a favorite grace together that gets us through the tough times. At other times it is a shared belief system that can build hope. In illnesses such as dementia, it is often long-term memory that keeps many of the religious and spiritual memories. Those with a religious tradition have a treasure store to draw from, and the congregation may assist families to unlock these remembrances.

Being aware of caregiver and care receiver feelings and walking alongside as they struggle are important parts of ministry. To be effective, people from the church need to listen with open minds and hearts.

5 Concerns about Abuse in the Caregiving Family

Although no one likes to think about it, the issue of elder abuse can be a concern in caregiving relationships. The church plays a vital role in prevention and education. Visitors to those who receive care should be aware of stressed caregivers and unusual situations, and raise warning flags if necessary but refrain from blaming or making decisions. The abused and abusers may be members of the church, and it is true that we are our brothers' and sisters' keepers.

Abuse is the mistreatment or neglect of a person. It can take many forms: physical, emotional/psychological, financial, and sexual. There are also situations of active or passive neglect in which a person is harmed. Abuse occurs on a continuum from less to more severe. Observance of sharp words spoken by the caregiver or unusual bruises on the care receiver should be red flags. These can simply be signs of heavy stresses in caregiving or they may be the warning signs of potential abuse. And they can be symptoms of a deteriorating situation.

Women, persons in poor health, those who are isolated, people on limited incomes, and those from age sixty to eighty-four are the most vulnerable to abuse. Intimate partners are the most apt to abuse, and sometimes there is a long history of abuse between partners. Sometimes the abuse is done by a stronger partner who had been abused at a time when he or she was more vulnerable. Adult children and adult children's spouses are also frequent abusers.

The abusers may have problems with substance abuse, mental or emotional illness, lack of caregiving experience, stress and burdens from financial difficulties, dependency, lack of social support, marital problems, or dementia.

Factors that can set up the possibility of abuse for victims include general ill health, impairments in the ability to do the tasks of life (bathing and eating for example), dependence on the abuser, isolation from others, and conflicted marital relationships over time. Caregivers run the risk of becoming abusers when they are providing care to several generations, experience lack of support or respite, struggle with personal psychosocial problems, have had a recent serious illness or loss, are dependent on the victim, (e.g., for a place to stay or financial support), are persons who experienced abuse as a child or spouse, or who have been recently abused by the care receiver. The environment of abuse includes financial difficulties, family violence, lack of social support, family disharmony, and living in close proximity.

There are many theories about abuse and many conditions under which it exists. For purposes here, it is important to look at concerns related to caregiving's stresses and strains. Learned behavior of abuse or family cycles of violence can bubble up again when an elder is disabled and vulnerable, added to the intense stress of day-to-day, hour-to-hour care. There are some warning signals that indicate when a caregiver might be at risk for some problems and possibly abuse. These include: (1) hiding feelings from others who could be supportive, (2) trying to be a superperson by doing it all, (3) having values, belief systems, and cultural imperatives about caring that get in the way of self-care, (4) lacking education about options for resources to alleviate stress, (5) isolation, (6) taking care receiver criticism too personally, (7) using alcohol or drugs to deaden problems, (8) worrying excessively about money, (9) worrying about several generations depending on the caregiver, (10) a long history of family dysfunction (especially one in which violence was a way to respond to stress), and (11) having family members at serious odds about caring. These all need serious consideration.

Those who support caregivers should be aware of these issues. A person can then gently check out how the person is doing emotionally. Caregivers may not ask for help because of shame or because they do not know there are services that could lighten their stress and burden.

Prevention is important. Being able to vent one's feelings in an appropriate way to a safe person (such as clergy) can decrease the possibility of abuse. Linking with agencies to provide in-home services can be useful. Support groups can be helpful because the caregiver can share similar concerns without judgment. Respite care is crucial. Education about dealing with feelings that could become abusive can be valuable. Caregivers and receivers alike may need support. The overstressed caregiver needs encouragement to use services. Issues of guilt and shame that often accompany elder abuse need to be openly discussed. Caregivers may need assistance in contingency planning for future situations. The church can play a vital role by being aware of resources and helping others to connect with them. If a dangerous situation is in place, the visitor may need to call Adult Protective Services. It is important that all in the community of faith remember that they do not have to prove abuse. The professionals in the community have that responsibility. It is important to find out the reporting requirements in the state. An elder's life may depend on it. Although it is distasteful to think about, people in the church cannot wish away the existence of abuse.

6   Ethical and Spiritual Issues

Many concerns faced by families involve ethical and spiritual dilemmas. Caregivers struggling with these concerns could benefit from sorting out all perspectives arising from their quandaries. The following delineation of the issues is adapted from an article by Pratt, Schmall, and Wright (1987).

Family caregiving responsibility relates to the difficult task of balancing needs of all family members. Each generation has its own, often conflicting, issues. Those in their middle years may be dealing with frail parents and grandparents, in addition to handling problems with children and grandchildren, and as a result can feel caught in the middle. This is the reason why they have been called the "sandwich generation" in the popular press. How does one decide where primary loyalty rests? What are the factors that go into that decision? How does one make difficult choices? There are no universal easy answers, but the community of faith should be responsive to caregivers' questions. The church could provide the crucible for debate.

Mutuality of moral obligations refers to reciprocity between generations. These dilemmas are often posed by questions about what is owed between family members. A daughter might ask, "If my mother took care of me when

I was a child, what shall I do for her now that she is frail?" Mutual respect is key. In the Jewish and Christian traditions, these messages of obligation are clearly outlined in the Ten Commandments. Other religious traditions have similar precepts ("filial piety" in Eastern traditions for example). But at the same time that caregivers reflect on such expectations in their heads and in their hearts, there is the reality that one cannot get water out of a dry well or blood out of a turnip. So each family must determine for itself where the limits of mutual respect lie for them.

Past issues unresolved illustrates the impact of family secrets. These can return to the family's consciousness to haunt both caregivers and receivers. If a person has struggled with such issues over a lifetime with parents or partners, how do they move forward to be caregivers? Secrets hidden for many years can rear their heads in a caregiving crisis. The child of a formerly alcoholic mother may find it difficult to care for her if she were to suffer a stroke. Even if that person has been sober and has changed in their later years, the issues of the past can be big barriers. The hurts of childhood memories can get in the way, and members of that family might need to come to grips with these pains. There is always the potential for forgiveness. However, forgiveness work takes time and there is no quick fix. Often there is the need for some intense counseling and pastoral support in order to work through the past.

The unfairness of God for allowing suffering is something many caregivers struggle with. Their faith is sorely tested. There can be issues of survivor guilt and quandaries about one's basic belief systems. They may question how God can let bad things happen to good people. The church can support families by listening carefully and reframing such concerns in terms of what is known about a particular illness or condition. Care must be taken not to take away the tenets of the caregiver's belief system, even when they seem judgmental. Caregivers need to hear the gospel messages of love and compassion. Persons from the church community can speak and role model these.

Issues regarding quality of life create other dilemmas. Quality of life can mean different things, but it generally relates to a good standard of living for a person, physically, mentally, emotionally, and spiritually. Each person has his or her own definition of this term, and caregivers and care receivers may see it differently. Working out quality-of-life differences is a balancing act for all. Persons who visit caregivers and receivers must use care not to judge a situation one way or another through their own filters and life experiences. The reality of a situation may be quite different from what one superficially encounters.

Making the best of worst choices is a dilemma caregivers deal with when faced with the problem of independence versus care. Sometimes what is the best option for an elder becomes problematic for the whole system. All in the family need to honestly evaluate choices in light of what is best for each member. For example, most disabled people would choose to live at home with as much independence as possible. However, there are times when caregiver exhaustion or care receiver safety issues may need to be considered more urgently than that push for independence. A person may need institutional care rather than home care. Other concerns include questions about an acceptable level of safety risk, and when to allow a person to fail. Choices for using outside help or long-term care facility placement may need to be made.

As families struggle with choices, they can benefit from talking about them with someone from the faith community. Whatever resource concerns get raised, and whatever choices are made, need to be honestly shared with the care receiver in a way that he or she can understand. Older adults are more willing to accept services if families are honest about the considerations surrounding the choices. Families are sometimes reluctant to be honest out of a misguided fear of hurting their loved one, and in the long run this makes matters worse. And it must be stated here that families are still caregivers when someone goes to a long-term care facility. They have not failed in their role. Some have reported that the relationship with their loved one has improved when they were able to relinquish some of the heavy-duty tasks of caregiving.

Strengths and pitfalls of technology are the issues at the basic core of caring. Today's technology is complex and more readily available than ever before. Families deal with questions today not dreamed of back when people routinely died of pneumonia. And simple technological devices such as lifeline and improved hearing aids enable elders to keep in touch with others. Technological decisions about caring (life supports, for example) need to be thought through. Questions about when to treat a person with Alzheimer's disease aggressively is an example of the modern struggle with technology. Some basic questions can be raised. When is enough treatment enough? What resources should be used? Is there a limit to these? Where is there a sense of justice between all generations? There are no easy answers. The questions *do* inform the way that caregiving is provided. And larger policy issues and laws play their part in the discussions as well.

Safety vs. autonomy is another set of dilemmas revolving around decisions concerning when to protect a person and when to allow that person to fail. It is important for care receivers to do as much as they can for themselves. However, there are times when there must be limits imposed on independence. Caregivers must guard against smothering, or doing something for a person that he or she could do alone. This is true even for the little things in life. The dignity of a care receiver needs affirmation at all times, and assisting a person to be safely independent is part of this.

The following is a process that could aid caregivers working through ethical issues, but this is not a cookbook of solutions. These steps could be worked through in a pastoral care situation, with the parish nurse, or by a referral to a health or social services professional.

First, identify the problems and the strengths in a situation. Coming to a common understanding of what the problems are goes a long way toward coping with them.

Definition is not an easy task, as everyone involved may have a different perspective.

Second, clarify the concerns of all, including the caregiver, care receiver, agencies, and others involved. People in the community of faith might be part of this. Some values that may be involved are independence (autonomy), safety, a need to be in control, and acting in the best interests of all.

Third, identify all options and outcomes available. The pros and cons of each should be clearly defined. Writing these out is often helpful.

Only after going through these steps can a realistic option be chosen. There is the tendency to want to cut short this process and, as a result, plans fail over time. The choice should be one that all involved can accept. This decision may in fact represent the best of the worst choices, or it may be a compromise where everyone has had to give in on some points. Reaching consensus in dealing with a concern is a necessary process, but it does not come easily.

After carefully examining the problem and the values involved and choosing an option, a choice can be made. Monitoring the results and reflecting on the decision is key. Changes can be made if necessary, as nothing is cast in concrete.

The following questions might be raised in working through this process: What is owed between generations in a family? How is money spent for care? The answers to these questions may inform how care is given and who in the family might be identified as a caregiver. The needs of both caregiver and care receiver as well as the values that inform each person can be carefully evaluated. The following worksheet might be used by families to sort out the issues in their caregiving situation.

7   A Worksheet for Caregivers

Remember there is no one right answer for every situation. You need to do the best that you can do for your concerns.

What is the situation in which you find yourself?

What is your loved one's diagnosis? What is his or her functional ability? (needs assistance with dressing, belligerent)

What are your loved one's needs? (emotional, physical, mental, spiritual) (safe environment, someone to deal with behavioral concerns, stimulation/communication)

What is the decision that needs to be made? (moving to a care facility)

What are your needs? (emotional, physical, mental, spiritual) (knowledge that loved one is cared for, sleep, peace of mind, understanding behavioral issues)

What is your financial situation? (limited dollars, social security)

Other things to consider specific to your situation:

What are the options (choices) available to you?

What are the values behind your decision-making process? Where did they come from? (the church, society, family)

Who can you turn to for help? (clergy, counselors)

What community agencies can assist you? Where are they? What needs are there for planning ahead? (adult family homes, adult daycare, assisted living, nursing homes)

Is there help available from the church? (minister, parish nurse)

What books, tapes, or videos might be helpful?

What are the consequences of the various options? (pros and cons of each option for your loved one and for you)

What are the benefits of the various options? (peace of mind, a sense of doing all that you could, family harmony)

What are the costs? (financial and emotional)

How much risk are you willing to take on? (bounded choices)

How much guilt can you live with? (It will always be with you to some extent—how much can you live with?)

8   Communication Strategies

When caregivers and care receivers live together, honest communication is important. All too often families push feelings under the surface, and those feelings later come out and upset everyone. Or those feelings stay inside and depression is the result. Obviously emotions need to be shared in ways that are constructive and understandable to others. For care receivers, the ability to comprehend can be affected by dementia or other illness processes. Sensory losses need to be taken into account when sharing communications. What is being said on the surface (fact/content) may not be what is really going on (feeling/process). Both fact and feeling are part of communication and need to be heard. Good communication is a way of sharing love.

Here are some specific ways to open dialogue between caregiver and care receiver: (1) Have information about concerns and resource knowledge available before sharing with a loved one. (2) Be sensitive to all losses faced by an elder. (3) Put issues in terms of a carer's requirement to know for planning, so that an elder doesn't feel his or her privacy is being invaded. (4) Remember that the person cared for is an adult even when dependent on others. (5) Give as many choices as realistically possible, allowing control even in small things. (6) Build on the continuity of an elder's strengths. (7) Ask for third-party assistance when there are blocks in communication.

The congregation can assist families in learning such communication skills in educational classes or support groups. Through pastoral care, parish nurse visits, and lay support, the church can model communication skills. This can be done primarily by listening to both the caregiver and the care receiver, and treating what each has to say as important.

9 Long-Distance Caregiving

Long-distance caregivers are important. As persons move about in this mobile society, concerns for a loved one may be intensified. Yet long-distance caring may not always be acknowledged. People at a distance do offer support and encouragement, and sometimes financial assistance. The caregiving may take a different form, but it is caregiving all the same. Modern communication has made it possible to keep in close contact with those being cared for by telephone and, in more recent times, via e-mail.

When there is a live-in caregiver, the long-distance person can make reassuring phone calls, make respite visits, and give general appreciation for what a caregiver is doing. A problem can exist when perceptions differ between those who see someone daily and those who visit infrequently. Those at a distance may feel that the caregiver is exaggerating problems. Or they may be shocked at their loved one's appearance because the caregiver has minimized a condition. Friction can occur when a care receiver praises the out-of-town person and picks on the day-to-day caregiver. The person at a distance should remember that he or she is there only for a short time and could appear to be a white knight to the disabled person. Therefore, the long-distance person should be sensitive to the person who gives the bulk of care and praise his or her efforts.

At times it may appear to an out-of-town person that decisions have been made in a capricious fashion. The reality is that the options chosen may have arisen out of a series of little compromises over time. Another complication in long-distance situations is that those receiving care may rise to the occasion of a visit by an out-of-town relative, so they may seem better than they really are. This can cloud reality for everyone involved, but especially for the person who has come in from out of town.

Usually out-of-town caregivers do not do hands-on work with their disabled relative. Questions may arise about where a disabled person should live, with which child, and in which city. An adult child may ponder whether to move home to become a caregiver; such a move might require leaving a job or family for an extended period. Families answer these questions in a variety of ways and there is no one right answer. Keeping track of someone is a concern, and some families may hire a private case manager to become their eyes and ears. They might make a pact with neighbors or friends to check in periodically. Another possibility might be to keep in touch with a person's church. Communities of faith could be very helpful in helping those with no family nearby by setting up a regular check-in time and then communicating with the long-distance family members about their loved one's situation.

Out-of-town caregivers can benefit from counseling and support. When they visit their loved one, it is important that they keep their own support networks intact. Because many use vacation time to check on out-of-town elders, they need to remember to take time out for themselves as well. If they are planning to contact local resources, it is wise to call ahead so that appropriate help can be available during the short time of their visit.

In exhaustion and frustration, some family members seek to move a loved one closer to themselves. This needs to be looked at very carefully. Clear boundaries about what can and cannot be done must be determined. Moving to a new community may mean separation from another network of support other than family members (the church, neighbors, and others). Even the weather and way of life can be so radically different as to create problems. Out-of-town carers in different cities may not support each other in decision making and this can add another level of stress. A family conference with all involved via telephone or in person can go a long way to clear the air. Such a meeting can also set up a plan of care for a care receiver, including what each person can do to execute parts of the plan. Writing out the plan for all to have can be useful.

Lustbader and Hooyman in *Taking Care* (1994, p. 106) and others offer some tips for keeping in contact with out-of-town elders. These suggestions include: (1) making regular phone calls, and having an extension if there are two people (one might also encourage elders to call collect, or give telephone time gift certificates); (2) writing frequent newsy letters, sending video or audio tapes and newspaper clippings of family activities or even postcards with simple messages, or sending e-mail messages if that capability exists; (3) providing return-address labels and pre-addressed stamped envelopes, as some elders are uncomfortable about their writing ability; (4) giving a box of all-occasion greeting cards so that an older person can remember people on special days; (5) keeping a phone book and/or senior resource directory from the city where a loved one lives handy to the phone and; (6) connecting to long-distance care networks (such as ElderCare Locator) to find resources for a loved one.

10   Empowering Caregivers for Self-Care

Families caring for someone with a disability may put all of their energy into their loved one's care at the expense of their own health and well-being. It is ironic that at the very time when caregivers might benefit from the concern of the church, they may be most apt to pull back. Members of the community of faith need to be sensitive to that. And people in the church may not know how to most effectively reach out to those who might benefit from such support. They may need assistance from a specialist on aging for some suggestions about the best ways to offer assistance. There is a fine line that the community of faith walks between being helpful and interfering.

There are some things that caregivers can do to empower themselves and to ultimately better the situation for themselves and the person they care for.

1. It is important to help caregivers learn all they can about options, resources, and community assistance. Looking at the pros and cons of each possibility for help and writing them down can often give a clear picture of what is happening. When one gets clear information and choices, it can help in decreasing the sense of being overwhelmed. The congregation might provide a resource bank and a lending library of books and materials.

2. Give caregivers permission to ask for help. All in the church need to remember this, even when it is most obvious that help is required in caregiving. Caregivers cannot be all things to all people, no matter how hard they try. Pastoral counselors, Stephen ministers, and parish nurses can remind people about this.

3. Encourage people to plan ahead. This can be emotionally difficult because people have to look at their own vulnerabilities. It is important to do contingency planning when thinking about the future. Something as basic as planning which neighbor to call in an emergency can be reassuring. Knowing that a plan is in place, even if it is never utilized, is a source of comfort for stressed-out caregivers. Classes about caregiving or advanced directives and other issues can be facilitated to aid people in planning.

4. Provide opportunities for caregivers to interact with others at educational sessions and support groups. Finding out they are not alone in the journey can be of great help. Offering respite for a care receiver can often enable a caregiver to attend a meeting. People from the church might also offer to attend such sessions with a caregiver.

5. Help caregivers learn to advocate for their rights and the rights of the person they care for. Persons may need encouragement to be empowered about such rights. These rights are especially important as people deal with the social and healthcare systems where they may feel overwhelmed by paperwork and red tape.

6. Caregivers need to be honest with themselves about what they realistically can and can't do. Each person is

unique and has different breaking points. While someone who goes the second or third mile in caregiving gets admiration and affirmation, it is also necessary to be aware of caregivers who are approaching burnout and could benefit from talking through their issues.

7. Caregivers do not have to do it all alone. Families need to evaluate what their whole network can do to provide for a disabled person. This takes honest assessment and a willingness to reach out to others. Hands-on caregivers can share the difficult tasks and the joys with others by honestly speaking to their needs. And the church can be ready with assistance when it is appropriate to improve the quality of life for a person.

11 Learning to Use Resources

Even when caregivers are trying as hard as they can to do a good job, they can exhaust their own resources in time, energy, and money. There comes a time when they may benefit from receiving services from community social and health agencies. As noted previously, it can be very difficult to ask for assistance when one is used to feeling totally independent. There are fears of others being a part of one's day-to-day life, and every time there is a negative story about community services in the media, the fears are exacerbated.

Every community has some services for elders and the disabled and their caregivers; however, not all resources are available in every community. A few examples are illustrative here. In adult daycare programs, persons go a few hours a day for socialization, meals, and activities while the caregiver benefits from some time out. Home health services include those that can assist with activities of daily living (bathing or dressing, for example), household tasks (cooking or shopping), and other jobs. Hospice can provide pain management and support to a person who is dying at home. There are many other services as well.

These services can usually be contacted through a main number for area agencies on aging. They might be called Senior Information and Assistance, or Services to Seniors, or some similar name. Throughout the country, these information lines can be the starting point for finding assistance. Remember that there are no easy answers to problems, so persons may have to talk with more than one service. Also, there may be some limits to eligibility based on income or care needs. Some are free, some require a co-payment, some may be offered on a sliding fee scale, and still others may require a total payment. Caregivers can become frustrated when the first agency they call is not able to answer all the questions or deal with every problem. The church might be able to help with this process by having a general sense of what the resources in a community are and offering to assist a caregiver in tracking down information, or by going to an appointment with the caregiver to enable him or her to connect with those things that are needed.

Some helpful suggestions for calling agencies are offered in the *Memphis Interfaith Association's Resource Guide: Caring Is a Family Affair* (1998, p. 18) and adapted here. In order to have the best success when calling agencies:

1. Organize the facts of the situation. Know the questions where answers are needed. Be as clear as possible on the call, since having to call back can be difficult and time consuming. Ask about costs involved for services.
2. Be as specific as possible in presenting the needs for services. This will be helpful to the person screening the call.
3. Call in the morning hours. There is a better chance

of catching workers then, and they will have had fewer crises to deal with at that time.

4. Keep notes on the call. Note the name of the worker, the date, time, and information shared. This may be relevant at the time and also later.

5. Be assertive. If there are difficulties, ask about a better time to call back, or ask to speak with a supervisor.

6. Remember to say thank you. These basic tips for arranging services can make the process less stressful.

12   Building on Hope

Christians are people of hope. Remembering the Easter message keeps many going throughout their lives. Caregivers and care receivers need hope in their caring as well. They face transitions and changes of many kinds, as Kathy Fischer reminds us in *Autumn Gospel* (1996):

> Faith tells us that this circle of loss and gain is a crucible of transformation. It is the paradox of the Gospel: if you want to keep your life, give it away. A seed must die to bring forth fruit. During the immense struggle to embrace loss and change, what we need most is hope, the trust that if we loosen our grip on the old, we will still have something. Part of this hope is being able to understand in faith the pattern of transitions: the ending, the period in-between and the emergence of something new. Each stage has its characteristic challenges and graces.

And indeed the changes and losses in caregiver relationships require a sense of hope.

Some very interesting work on hope has come out of the work of Farran, Herth, and Popovich (1995), who have studied this idea as it relates to illness and health. Their concept of hope and health can be helpful to caregivers and those who support them. They define the attributes of hope in the following ways: (1) as an experiential process;

(2) as a spiritual or transcendent process; (3) as a rational thought process; and (4) as a relational process.

Each of these has implications for caregivers. In studying hope as an experiential process, one can see that part of this relates to accepting a chronic illness or suffering as part of oneself. It helps when one can see that the boundaries of the possible are greater than the limits of the impossible. When one can have small successes, or solve small problems, it can have great meaning in the caregiving situation and can offer hope.

In considering hope as a spiritual process, it becomes clear that for many hope is inseparable from their faith or religious outlook. For Christians, even in the dark days of being a care receiver or caregiver, there is the strong message coming through that God will walk with them through the situation, and that there is a better world to come in the afterlife. In a helpful meditation book for caregivers to those with Alzheimer's disease (Murphey, 1988, p. 109), a caregiver recounts: "I'm enjoying life more as I appreciate again these simple things we have around us all the time."

The construct of hope as a rational thought process offers much as communities of faith seek to aid caregivers. As Ferran and her colleagues outline their thoughts, there are five parts to hope as a rational thought process. To have hope one needs to have *goals*—something to work toward. A simple example of this can be seen when, after months of rehabilitation, a person can button his or her shirt again without having to depend on others to do it.

There might be emotional goals as well. *Resources*, which can be internal or external, are also part of hope. A sense of humor is an internal resource; financial security is an external resource. Hope is seen as an *active process*. People are involved in doing something about their lives; life is not done to them. *Control* over one's destiny is another aspect of this. Helping care receivers to do as much as they can is part of this; disability often robs from ability. Control can bring back hope. People need *time* to struggle with relationships, work on rehabilitation, and pull together life's meanings. Time is needed to cope and to adapt to doing something a new way after a stroke. The church can help both caregivers and care receivers to work on hope as a rational thought process of setting goals, offering resources, helping with the active process, giving control to the care receiver, and taking the time to be present for both caregiver and receiver.

One of the most important parts of exploring hope is looking at it as a relational process. There are many things about caregiving that can't be changed. However, knowing that someone is there to walk beside you in the struggles goes a long way in maintaining hope. Standing shoulder to shoulder assists in strengthening persons when standing alone can be too difficult. The congregation's members can offer hope through their presence to those walking the caregiving road. Hope is realistic; it is not denial or an overly positive way of seeing the world. It is important for the well-being of all in the caregiving situation. The church has an important role in maintaining hope for caregivers and receivers.

Hope is also a factor as one grieves. Grief needs to be processed before things seem normal again. It is important that helpers don't try to dry the tears too soon, as there needs to be a chance to express catharsis through those tears. Again, the faith community can stand by someone as they go through a grief process.

To maintain a sense of hope, caregivers need to practice whatever spiritual disciplines they have used throughout their lives. These include praying and meditating, reading the scripture, singing, using ritual and symbol, healing services, and visual arts. Some congregations have offered caregiver retreats for renewal and assistance in exploring those disciplines again in new ways.

Hope also is related to humor. Over and over, caregivers note that it is the ability to laugh, to see the absurd, or to take themselves lightly that keeps them going. It is a survival skill that allows people to stay flexible and fluid in their world view. The writer knew this when he stated in Proverbs 17:22, "A cheerful heart is a good medicine, but a downcast spirit dries up the bones." All in the caregiving situation need not dry out.

There is hope in the survival of the human spirit for both caregivers and care receivers. Those who are helpers can be learners and gain a great deal. Hands-on caregivers often have creative solutions for concerns that had seemed very difficult. There can be hope in helping others understand caregiving roles.

13   What the Church
       Can Do to Help

There are many practical things that a congregation can do to assist caregivers in its midst. Although every congregation is unique and every caregiving concern is different, there are some things that the church can do to help. A few ideas are offered here, but it is important to remember that there is no template that fits every situation. Sometimes congregations need to be aware of opportunities to join with churches of their own and other traditions to share resources and creativity. And linking with community agencies can be useful. Many of these ideas are adapted from the work of Elaine Tiller.

1. A very basic core philosophy for being with those in a caregiving situation is to continue remembering both the caregiver and the care receiver in prayer, as both need spiritual support. One caregiver poignantly recounted her frustrations with well-meaning friends who would always ask about her husband. She cried out: "Just once I wish someone would ask how I am doing!" For Christians, the thought that someone remembers them in prayer can be a source of great comfort and strength. One congregation has special prayers for the homebound one Sunday per month on a regular basis.

2. Churches need to consult with those actually in the caregiving role about what would be helpful for them. They have much to teach about love, survival, and caring. Don't make assumptions about what caregivers feel. One woman wanted her pastor to understand her dilemmas in dealing with her husband's dementia. When it was suggested that she might share her concerns with him, her immediate response was, "Oh, he wouldn't understand." Caregivers need to feel that their issues will be heard. Churches can assist people in the caring role by listening and trying to understand their stories.

Caregivers may need help with self-care. The idea of caring for oneself is often thought of as selfishness by caregivers. This may need to be reframed as helping their loved one by caring for themselves. Persons in the faith community then become permission givers in encouraging such self-care. People from the church can also learn to recognize the red flags of stress in order to prevent abuse. These persons may also be trained to learn symptoms of abuse and how to properly report their suspicions to the authorities.

3. Examples of family dilemmas and Christian life are often shared from the pulpit. Using examples of what it means to be a caregiver can be a powerful message to someone in that role that the faith community is tuned in to their needs. It says someone here understands my situation. This can help alleviate some of the loneliness caregivers describe.

4. Congregations can train volunteers to be visitors and advocates for elders who find themselves in healthcare systems, since being in those places may be a scary experience for elders and their carers. Having someone to walk that path with them can be very reassuring.

5. Many churches have a commissioned parish nurse or health minister. Some have nurses serving in a volunteer role, or in conjunction with a local hospital. This person can make a bridge between the physical health, mental health, and spiritual aspects of life for all. He or she can provide special support to elders and their families. In many churches the parish nurse coordinates health fairs, health education, blood pressure checks, and health department immunization days.

6. Having volunteers who can give tangible assistance in shopping, cleaning, cooking, or respite care to a caregiving family may make the difference in a caregiver's ability to continue in his or her role. National Interfaith Caregivers have programs throughout the country where collaboration among several congregations has provided needed community services to the disabled and special-needs persons of all ages.

7. Some groups have formalized Stephen Ministry or other structured ministry programs. These lay ministers have been lifelines to many caregivers. Training in this program provides good information about a variety of topics including helping the elderly and their families and setting appropriate boundaries for sharing. Issues that

might be dealt with include guilt and decision making, building family relationships, and looking at the value systems of those giving care. Such a program also provides support to the volunteers through regular supervision.

8. A very useful service provided by some church groups is having a loan program of hospital or durable equipment that caregivers and care receivers can draw from as needed. This is not only a convenience but can help caregivers financially as well.

9. Some congregations have instituted a regular check-in calls program. During these calls, the person on the phone should ask about both caregiver and care receiver. This gives the message to the homebound that the community of faith cares about them.

10. Regular visits from a pastoral team are also important to those facing caregiving. Visitors should phone ahead and let people know they are coming. Plan for times convenient to the care routine. During those visits the life of the congregation might be shared by bringing bulletins, tapes of the Sunday service, and other special events. Visitors can also encourage caregivers and receivers alike to share feelings and memories about their life in the church. Tangibly bringing congregational life to those homebound can offer a real sense that they are not forgotten.

11. One of the most important things a congregation can do is use education as a tool to help caregivers. All in the congregation can benefit from such education, not just those who are caregivers now or plan to be caregivers in the future. Educational opportunities can be offered dur-

ing the regular adult education hour or at special times convenient for caregivers. Provide respite care to the ill person so that a caregiver might attend a class.

Some of the topics that could be discussed include: (1) planning for the future (advance directives, funeral plans, and legal planning, for example), (2) specific illness processes and how to help people who struggle with them (dealing with dementia is an often-requested topic), (3) relationship changes in aging families, especially those in the caregiving role, (4) basic care issues such as nutrition, lifting, and transferring, (5) how to access and use resources, and (6) meeting the spiritual needs of persons struggling with ill health.

Persons from outside resources could provide classes on what is available in the community. If there is a church-sponsored long-term care facility nearby, find out if it has speakers available who could talk about some of these issues.

12. Having an accessible resource file of community services has been of help in many congregations. This can be available to caregivers and to all in volunteer and staff positions who might encounter a person in need of information. The person who initially answers the phone at the church should be especially encouraged to have that resource file available or know how to refer people with questions to someone in the congregation who has a grasp of the information. Some congregations have sponsored resource/health fairs where agencies bring materials and share what they do. Other groups have a resource bulletin

board highlighting particular programs. Services that could be highlighted include adult daycare, respite care, support groups, and area agency-on-aging programs.

13. The congregational newsletter can be a place for articles about resources and caregiving issues as well. Just a small column written by the parish nurse, other staff member, or volunteer can help those at home know that others are aware of their situation. And the information will reach them even when they are homebound.

14. Having books and pamphlets in the church library about caregiving and coping with disability can be very useful. Consider also having books for children that tell stories about elders with particular concerns. The Alzheimer's Association and other agencies often have material that could be very valuable to caregivers.

15. Churches can sponsor and/or be a place where support groups meet. These can focus on caregiving in general or on a particular concern (stroke or Alzheimer's disease for example).

16. Church members benefit from information about public policy and legislative efforts that affect them and caregivers now and in the future. Issues about Medicare and other healthcare concerns are particularly sensitive. People of all generations need to be aware of these issues. They can be discussed not only in terms of the practical information about how legislation will affect individuals, but also in terms of bigger justice issues.

17. Some congregations have instituted transportation programs to assist caregivers and receivers in getting to

church services, doctor's appointments, and other places. This has been a most helpful service. Transportation is a major issue for many, and the lack of such help can increase isolation.

18. Adult daycare programs where care receivers go for a few hours each day are important for providing respite. Some churches have developed such programs by themselves, others in conjunction with other churches or community agencies. It may be useful to provide such a program.

19. Giving a caregiver some time away is a great gift. Some groups have offered respite. One woman caring for a husband with Alzheimer's disease noted: "My church gives me Thursday nights. For four hours they sit with my husband and I can do anything I want. I have gotten my life back."

20. Another idea for congregations helping caregiving families is to provide a central filing system to maintain records about funeral plans, healthcare decisions, and other matters. The minister can work with families on all of these issues.

21. Congregations can also assist long-distance caregivers by keeping in touch with their in-town loved one and letting the person know how the congregant is doing. Churches can be part of the network to help those at a distance and can also be a referral source.

Obviously, everything on such a list of ideas will not fit the abilities of a particular congregation. Hopefully there may be other churches with which to work. And collaborating with community agencies can be very helpful. It takes creativity to figure out how to do that.

Closing Thoughts

Stephen Sapp's *When Alzheimer's Disease Strikes* (1996, pp. 49–50) is a helpful book for those who care for people with Alzheimer's disease. He shares some ideas about the positive aspects of caregiving that can serve as a way to close this book. His points are well taken for those who are caregivers to persons with many difficulties. He notes that caregivers mention the following as some of the rewards in the caregiving struggle: (1) knowing that one has fulfilled the obligation to honor a parent or stay faithful to a marriage vow; (2) understanding that one has done a difficult job well; (3) learning that one can do things one had never attempted before; (4) gaining a new closeness in the family as all work together to help a loved one; (5) renewing a sense of wonder in seeing the world through the eyes of their impaired person; and most importantly, (6) increasing their sense of a closer relationship with God as God walks with them on their caregiving path.

All congregations can work to study and understand values about what it means to be dependent and independent in the context of the Christian tradition. Learning to give and receive help are gifts to and from caregivers and care receivers. Through study and looking at biblical models, churches can learn about these things. Caregiving is a relationship; one of many over a lifetime. Caring for one another comes from consideration of the common good. Be there for the caregiver. It is not the words that are said but the presence of the people in community of faith that counts. Bless the carer and the care receiver with the gift of assistance.

Resources

American Association of Retired Persons and Administration on Aging. *A Profile of Older Americans*. Washington, D.C.: AARP, 1997.

Farran, C. J., K. A. Herth, and J. M. Popovich. *Hope and Hopelessness: Critical Clinical Constructs*. Thousand Oaks, Calif.: Sage Publications, 1995.

Fischer, K. *Autumn Gospel: Women in the Second Half of Life*. New York: Paulist Press, 1996, 28–29.

Lustbader, W. *Counting on Kindness: The Dilemmas of Dependency*. New York: Free Press, 1994.

Lustbader, W., and N. Hooyman. *Taking Care of Aging Family Members*. New York: Free Press, 1994.

Mace, N., and R. Rabins. *The Thirty-six Hour Day*. Baltimore: Johns Hopkins University Press, 1991.

Memphis Interfaith Association. *MIFA Caregivers Resource Guide: Caring Is a Family Affair*. Memphis: MIFA, 1998. (MIFA, 910 Vance, Memphis, TN 38126.)

Murphey, C. *Day to Day: Spiritual Help When Someone You Love Has Alzheimer's*. Philadelphia: Westminster Press, 1988.

Pratt, C., V. Schmall, and S. Wright. "Ethical Concerns of Family Caregivers to Dementia Patients," *The Gerontologist* 27(5): 1987, 632–38.

Sapp, S. *When Alzheimer's Disease Strikes*. Palm Beach, Fla.: Desert Ministries, 1996. (Desert Ministries, Inc., P.O. Box 788, Palm Beach, FL 33480.)

Tiller, D. E. *20 Ways Your Congregation Can Support Caregivers and Carereceivers*. Washington, D.C.: Baptist Senior Adult Ministries, 1991. (202) 628-4924.

Alzheimer's Association (located in Chicago with local offices throughout the country), (800) 272-3900. Books and pamphlets on caregiving, especially for those who are caregivers to dementia patients.

Area Agencies on Aging (located throughout the country) have basic information and assistance for services to elder and disabled adults.

ElderCare Locator, (800) 677-1116. This national hotline number can assist in finding services for elders throughout the country. The ZIP code is needed for services to be accessed.

National Association of Private Care Managers, (520) 881-8008. This national group provides referrals to private case managers throughout the country.

National Federation of Interfaith Volunteer Caregivers, Inc., (914) 331-1358. This national group helps to set up programs for individual groups of churches providing caregiving services.